EMERGENCY FIRST AID GUIDE

Your Comprehensive Step by Step Guide to All Emergency Situations

Dr. Steve Ben

Copyright@2024

Table of Contents

CHAPTER ONE

Introduction to First Aid

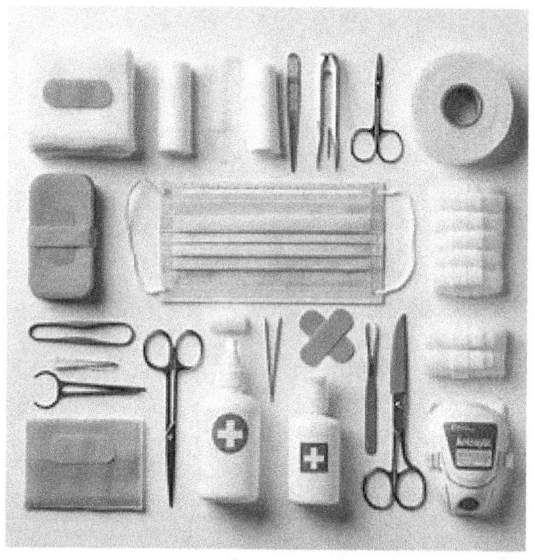

First aid refers to the immediate and initial assistance provided to individuals who have been injured or suddenly taken ill. It encompasses simple, life-saving techniques that can be performed with minimal equipment and training.

The importance of first aid lies in its ability to preserve life, prevent further harm, and promote recovery. Prompt and effective first aid interventions can significantly improve outcomes for the injured or ill person.

Legal Aspects and Good Samaritan Laws

Good Samaritan laws vary by jurisdiction but generally protect individuals who provide reasonable assistance to those who are injured or in peril, from being held liable for unintended consequences or injuries that may arise from their actions.

Understanding the legal aspects of first aid is essential for individuals providing assistance in emergency situations.

While these laws encourage people to help others in need, they also outline the boundaries and responsibilities of first aid providers.

Personal Safety Considerations

Before administering first aid, it's crucial to ensure personal safety. This involves assessing the scene for any potential hazards such as traffic, fire, or toxic substances.

Always prioritize your safety and the safety of others. If the scene is unsafe, wait for professional medical assistance to arrive before intervening.

Use personal protective equipment (PPE) such as gloves or face shields when providing first aid to reduce the risk of exposure to bloodborne pathogens or other bodily fluids.

Maintain awareness of your surroundings and be prepared to adapt to changing conditions while providing first aid.

By understanding the definition, importance, legal aspects, and personal safety considerations of first aid, individuals can be better prepared to respond effectively and responsibly in emergency situations, potentially saving lives and minimizing the impact of injuries or illnesses.

CHAPTER TWO

Assessment and Emergency Action

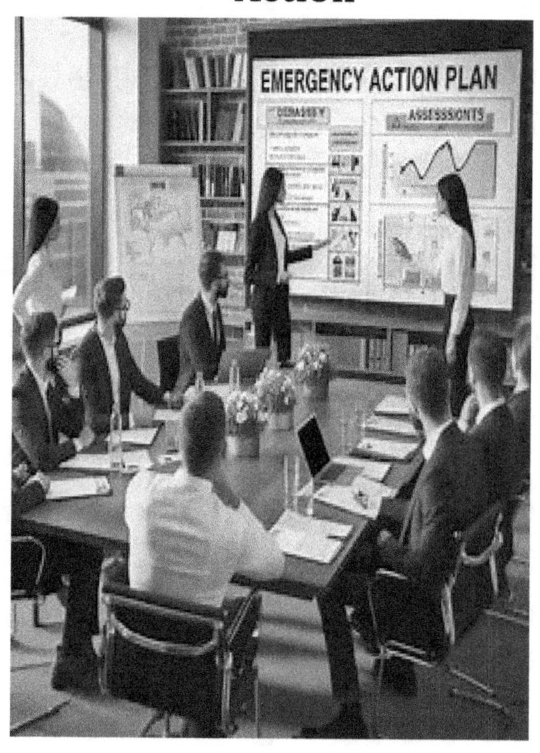

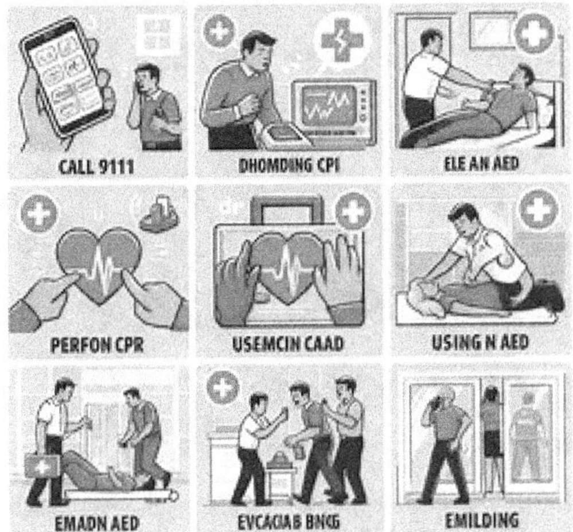

Scene Safety Assessment

Step 1: Initial Scene Survey

Instructs first responders to conduct a quick visual survey of the scene, identifying potential hazards such as fire, traffic, or hazardous materials.

Emphasizes the importance of ensuring personal safety before approaching the victim.

Step 2: Hazard Mitigation

Guides individuals on taking necessary steps to eliminate or minimize identified hazards, including moving to a safer location or notifying authorities.

Step 3: Ongoing Scene Monitoring

Stresses the need for continuous awareness of the surroundings to adapt to changing circumstances or additional risks.

Assessing the Victim's Level of Consciousness:

Step 1: Approach Safely

Teaches a cautious approach to the victim, ensuring the responder's safety and preventing further harm to the injured person.

Step 2: Stimulate and Assess Responsiveness

Instructs responders to gently tap and shout to check for a response, emphasizing the ABCs (Airway, Breathing, Circulation) throughout.

Step 3: Airway Assessment

Details the procedure for checking the victim's airway for obstructions, including the head-tilt, chin-lift maneuver.

Step 4: Breathing Assessment

Guides responders in observing chest rise and fall, listening for breath sounds, and feeling for airflow to determine breathing status.

Step 5: Circulation Assessment

Instructs individuals to check for signs of circulation, such as a pulse, and to assess for severe bleeding.

Basic Emergency Action Steps (Check-Call-Care):

Step 1: Check the Scene

Reinforces the importance of the initial scene assessment for safety and potential hazards.

Step 2: Call for Help

Guides individuals on making an emergency call, providing essential information such as the location, nature of the emergency, and the victim's condition.

Step 3: Care for the Victim

Teaches basic first aid interventions based on the victim's condition, such as providing CPR, managing bleeding, or stabilizing injuries until professional help arrives.

Step 4: Reassess the Victim

Emphasizes the need for ongoing reassessment, adapting care based on changes in the victim's condition or the arrival of professional medical assistance.

Special Considerations

Step 1: Pediatric Assessment

Addresses unique aspects of assessing and providing first aid to children, including modifications in techniques and considerations for age-appropriate care.

Step 2: Geriatric Assessment
Discusses considerations for assessing and assisting elderly individuals, highlighting potential challenges and adaptations in first aid approaches.

This detailed guide equips individuals with a structured approach to scene safety assessment, victim assessment, and the critical emergency action steps, providing a foundation for effective first aid interventions tailored to the specific needs of the situation.

CHAPTER THREE

Cardiopulmonary Resuscitation (CPR)

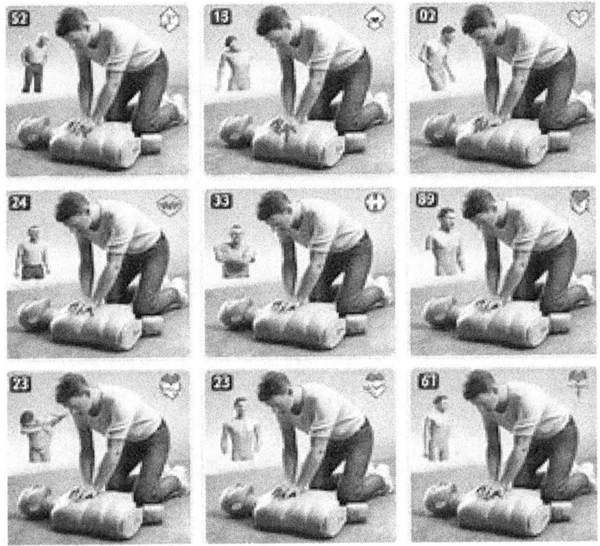

CPR Techniques for Adults, Children, and Infants:

1. Positioning and Preparation

Ensure the victim is lying on a firm, flat surface.

Assess the victim's responsiveness and breathing.

Call for emergency medical assistance if the victim is unresponsive or not breathing normally.

2. Adult CPR

Place the heel of one hand on the center of the victim's chest.

Place the other hand on top, interlocking the fingers.

Perform chest compressions at a rate of 100 to 120 compressions per minute, allowing the chest to fully recoil between compressions.

Administer rescue breaths, maintaining an open airway using the head-tilt, chin-lift maneuver.

3. Child and Infant CPR

Use two fingers for chest compressions in infants and the heel of one hand in children.

Modify the depth and force of compressions according to the size and age of the child.

Administer rescue breaths gently, covering the nose and mouth of the infant or child.

Use of Automated External Defibrillators (AEDs)

1. Assessing for AED Use

Check for the presence of an AED and retrieve it if available.

Turn on the AED and follow voice prompts or visual instructions.

2. Applying Electrodes

Remove clothing to expose the victim's chest.

Attach the AED pads to the victim's bare chest, following the placement instructions provided with the device.

3. Analyzing Heart Rhythm

Allow the AED to analyze the victim's heart rhythm.

Follow prompts to deliver a shock if advised by the device.

4. Resume CPR

After delivering a shock, immediately resume CPR, starting with chest compressions.

Hands-Only CPR versus Traditional CPR with Rescue Breaths:

1. Hands-Only CPR

Recommend hands-only CPR for untrained individuals or those uncomfortable with performing rescue breaths.

Emphasize the importance of continuous chest compressions at an appropriate rate until professional help arrives.

2. Traditional CPR with Rescue Breaths

Provide guidance on performing traditional CPR with rescue breaths for trained responders.

Stress the importance of maintaining an open airway and delivering effective rescue breaths.

Continuous Assessment and Reevaluation:

1. Monitor Response and Vital Signs

Continuously assess the victim's response to CPR interventions.

Check for signs of circulation, breathing, or responsiveness.

2. Reevaluate Interventions

Adjust CPR techniques and interventions based on changes in the victim's condition or the arrival of advanced medical support.

Special Considerations

1. Pregnant Victims: Provide guidance on modifying CPR techniques for pregnant victims while ensuring proper circulation and oxygenation.

2. Obese Victims: Address challenges and considerations for performing CPR on obese individuals, including optimal hand placement and compression depth.

This comprehensive approach to CPR equips individuals with the knowledge and skills needed to perform effective chest compressions, administer rescue breaths, and utilize AEDs in emergency situations involving adults, children, and infants. It also provides guidance on selecting the appropriate CPR technique based on the responder's level of training and comfort, along with continuous assessment and reevaluation to optimize patient outcomes.

CHAPTER FOUR

Choking Emergencies

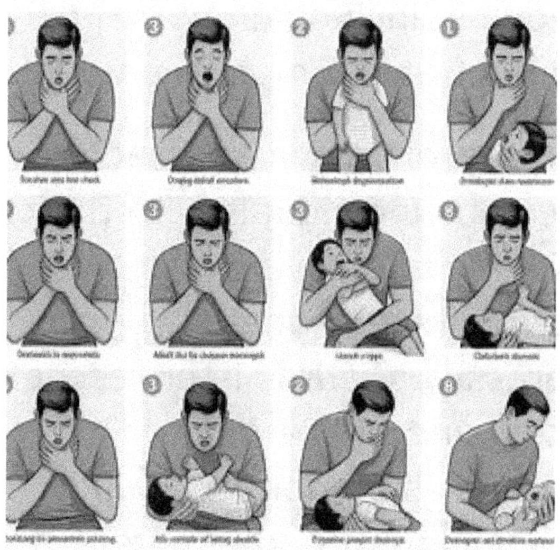

Recognizing Signs of Choking

Choking occurs when the airway is blocked, preventing normal breathing. It can happen when a foreign object, such as food or a small toy, becomes lodged in the throat.

Signs of choking may include;

-Clutching the throat

- Inability to speak or cough effectively

- Gasping for air

- Wheezing or high-pitched sounds while breathing

- Bluish discoloration of the lips, nails, or skin (cyanosis) in severe cases

- Prompt recognition of choking is crucial for timely intervention.

2. Performing Abdominal Thrusts (Heimlich Maneuver)

The Heimlich maneuver is a well-known technique used to dislodge an obstruction from the airway in conscious individuals.

- To perform the Heimlich maneuver

1. Stand behind the choking person and wrap your arms around their waist.

2. Make a fist with one hand and place the thumb side of the fist against the victim's abdomen, slightly above the navel and below the ribcage.

3. Grasp your fist with your other hand and press forcefully into the abdomen with a quick upward thrust.

4. Repeat abdominal thrusts until the object is dislodged or the victim becomes unconscious.

5. If the victim becomes unconscious, lower them gently to the ground and begin CPR, starting with chest compressions.

3. First Aid for Choking Victims Who Are Pregnant or Obese:

- Choking can present unique challenges in pregnant or obese individuals due to anatomical differences and changes in body shape.

- Modified techniques may be necessary to perform the Heimlich maneuver effectively.

- For pregnant individuals:

- Instead of placing the hands directly on the abdomen, use the chest thrust method by placing the hands at the base of the breastbone and delivering inward and upward thrusts.

- Avoid placing pressure on the abdomen to prevent injury to the uterus.

For obese individuals:

- Apply firm pressure to the abdomen with the heel of the hand while ensuring that the thrust is directed upward and inward.

- Adjust the position of the hands as needed to apply effective pressure and dislodge the obstruction.

- It's important to adapt the technique based on the individual's unique circumstances while prioritizing the safety and well-being of both the victim and the rescuer.

Recognizing the signs of choking and knowing how to perform the Heimlich maneuver effectively, individuals can respond promptly and decisively to choking emergencies, potentially preventing serious injury or even death. Understanding the modifications needed for pregnant or obese individuals enhances the responder's ability to provide appropriate first aid in diverse situations.

CHAPTER FIVE

Bleeding and Wound Care
Different Types of Bleeding (Arterial, Venous, Capillary)

Arterial bleeding occurs when blood is ejected from an artery. It is characterized by bright red blood that spurts rhythmically with each heartbeat.

Venous bleeding involves blood flowing from a vein. It tends to be steady and darker in color.

Capillary bleeding occurs from the smallest blood vessels and is characterized by oozing or slow bleeding.

Direct Pressure and Wound Care Techniques:

Direct pressure is the primary method for controlling bleeding in most cases.

To administer direct pressure:

1. Apply a clean cloth or sterile gauze directly over the wound.

2. Use your hand to apply firm pressure to the wound site.

3. Maintain pressure until bleeding stops or medical help arrives.

Elevating the injured area above the level of the heart can help reduce bleeding.

Avoid removing any objects that may be embedded in the wound, as they may be helping to control bleeding.

Once bleeding is controlled, clean the wound with mild soap and water to prevent infection.

Apply an appropriate dressing and secure it in place with bandages.

Use of Tourniquets and Hemostatic Agents:

Tourniquets are devices used to apply pressure to a limb to control bleeding in cases of severe hemorrhage.

When applying a tourniquet:

1. Place the tourniquet proximal (closer to the body) to the bleeding site.

2. Tighten the tourniquet until bleeding stops.

3. Secure the tourniquet in place and note the time of application.

4. Only use a tourniquet as a last resort when direct pressure fails to control bleeding or in cases of severe arterial bleeding.

Hemostatic agents are substances that promote blood clotting and can be used to control bleeding, particularly in cases of severe hemorrhage.

Apply hemostatic agents directly to the bleeding site and pack them into the wound if necessary.

Follow the manufacturer's instructions for the proper use of hemostatic agents.

It's important to assess the severity of bleeding and apply appropriate first aid measures accordingly.

Severe bleeding that is not controlled with direct pressure may require the use of tourniquets or hemostatic agents, but these measures should be used judiciously and with caution. Proper wound care techniques help prevent infection and promote healing. Additionally, seeking medical attention for severe bleeding is essential to address underlying causes and prevent complications.

CHAPTER SIX

Shock Management

Shock is a life-threatening condition characterized by inadequate blood flow and oxygen delivery to the body's tissues and organs.

Causes of shock may include severe injury, trauma, bleeding, dehydration, allergic reactions, heart failure, or severe infections.

Common symptoms of shock include:

- Pale, cool, clammy skin

- Rapid or weak pulse

- Rapid and shallow breathing

- Confusion or altered mental status

- Dizziness or fainting

- Nausea and vomiting

- Weakness or fatigue

2. First Aid Interventions to Manage Shock:

- If you suspect that someone is in shock, it's crucial to act quickly to stabilize their condition and prevent deterioration.

- Call emergency medical services (EMS) immediately and provide the dispatcher with essential information about the victim's condition and location.

- While waiting for help to arrive, follow these first aid interventions:

1. Lay the victim down on their back and elevate their legs about 12 inches unless they have a head, neck, or back injury.

2. Loosen tight clothing and cover the victim with a blanket or jacket to maintain body warmth.

3. Monitor the victim's airway, breathing, and circulation (ABCs) and be prepared to perform CPR if necessary.

4. Reassure the victim and keep them calm to reduce anxiety and stress.

5. Do not give the victim anything to eat or drink, as they may require emergency medical treatment.

Positioning and Comfort Measures for Shock Victims:

- Positioning the victim with elevated legs helps promote blood flow to vital organs, such as the heart and brain, by improving venous return.

- Ensure that the victim's head is in a neutral position to maintain proper alignment of the airway.

- Use pillows or rolled blankets to support the victim's legs in an elevated position, ensuring that they are comfortable and supported.

- Keep the victim warm to prevent further heat loss and maintain body temperature within a normal range.

- Avoid unnecessary movement or jostling of the victim to prevent exacerbating injuries or worsening their condition.

It's important to recognize the signs and symptoms of shock early and initiate prompt first aid interventions to prevent complications and improve outcomes.

While first aid measures can help stabilize the victim's condition temporarily, they should not replace definitive medical treatment provided by healthcare professionals. Shock management requires a coordinated effort between first responders, emergency medical services, and hospital personnel to ensure the best possible outcome for the victim.

CHAPTER SEVEN

**Burn Injuries
Classification of Burns (First, Second, Third Degree)**

First-degree burns: These burns affect only the outer layer of the skin (epidermis). They are characterized by redness, minor swelling, and pain. Sunburns are common examples of first-degree burns.

Second-degree burns: These burns affect both the outer layer of the skin (epidermis) and the underlying layer (dermis). They are characterized by blistering, severe pain, redness, and swelling.

Third-degree burns: These burns extend through all layers of the skin and may involve underlying tissues, muscles, and bones.

They often appear white, brown, or charred, and may be accompanied by numbness due to nerve damage.

Initial First Aid for Burns (Cooling, Covering, and Protecting the Area):

Cool the burn: Immediately after the burn occurs, run cool (not cold) water over the affected area for at least 10-20 minutes to help reduce pain, swelling, and further tissue damage. Avoid using ice or ice water, as it can cause additional damage to the skin.

Remove clothing and jewelry from the burned area, unless it is stuck to the skin. Clothing can retain heat and exacerbate the burn.

Cover the burn with a clean, dry cloth or sterile dressing to protect it from infection.

Avoid applying adhesive bandages directly to the burned area, as they may stick to the skin and cause further damage.

Avoid breaking blisters that may have formed, as they serve as a protective barrier against infection. However, if a blister breaks on its own, clean the area gently with mild soap and water and apply an antibiotic ointment.

Refrain from applying butter, oil, or other home remedies to the burn, as they can trap heat and increase the risk of infection.

Recognizing the Severity of Burns and When to Seek Medical Help:

Minor burns: First-degree burns and small second-degree burns that are less than 3 inches in diameter can often be treated at home with first aid measures.

However, if the burn covers a large area of the body, involves the face, hands, feet, or genitalia, or is accompanied by signs of infection (redness, swelling, pus), seek medical attention promptly.

Moderate to severe burns: Second-degree burns larger than 3 inches in diameter, third-degree burns, burns involving the face, hands, feet, or genitalia, and burns caused by chemicals, electricity, or inhalation should be evaluated by a healthcare professional immediately. These burns may require specialized treatment, such as debridement, skin grafting, or fluid resuscitation, to prevent complications and promote healing.

If the burn is caused by a chemical or electrical source, or if the victim is experiencing difficulty breathing, loss of consciousness, or signs of shock, call emergency medical services (EMS) immediately and provide appropriate first aid until help arrives. Understanding the classification of burns and administering appropriate first aid measures can help minimize pain, prevent complications, and promote healing. Recognizing the severity of burns and seeking medical help promptly is crucial for ensuring optimal outcomes and preventing long-term damage.

CHAPTER EIGHT

Musculoskeletal Injuries

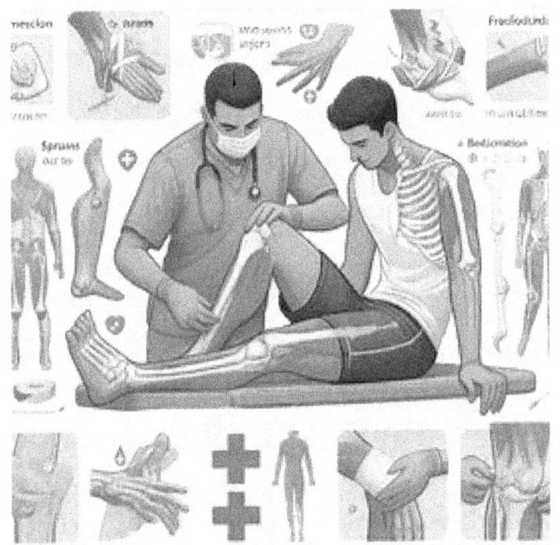

Assessing and Managing Fractures, Sprains, and Strains

Fractures: A fracture is a break in the continuity of bone tissue. Symptoms include pain, swelling, deformity, and difficulty moving the injured area.

To manage fractures, it's essential to immobilize the injured limb and seek medical attention promptly.

Sprains: Sprains occur when ligaments (tissues connecting bones) are stretched or torn. Symptoms include pain, swelling, bruising, and instability of the joint. Treatment involves rest, ice, compression, elevation (RICE), and sometimes physical therapy.

Strains: Strains involve stretched or torn muscles or tendons. Symptoms include pain, swelling, muscle spasm, and limited range of motion. Treatment also includes RICE therapy and gradual rehabilitation exercises.

Splinting Techniques for Different Body Parts

- Upper Extremity Splinting:

1. For forearm fractures: Place a rigid object (e.g., magazine, board) along the length of the forearm and secure it with bandages or cloth strips.

2. For wrist or hand injuries: Use a splint that immobilizes the wrist and hand in a neutral position.

Lower Extremity Splinting:

1. For leg fractures: Splint the injured leg to the uninjured leg to prevent movement. Use padding and bandages to secure the splint in place.

2. For ankle injuries: Use a splint that immobilizes the ankle and foot in a neutral position.

Spinal Immobilization:

1. If a spinal injury is suspected, maintain the victim's head, neck, and spine in a neutral position and avoid moving them unnecessarily.

2. Use a rigid cervical collar or improvised stabilization device (e.g., rolled towels) to support the neck and prevent movement.

3. Transport Considerations for Victims with Musculoskeletal Injuries:

Before moving the victim, assess their condition and immobilize any suspected fractures or spinal injuries.

If possible, use a stretcher or backboard to transport the victim to minimize movement and prevent further injury.

Enlist the help of bystanders or emergency responders to assist with lifting and transporting the victim safely.

Avoid dragging or twisting the victim's body during transport, as this can exacerbate musculoskeletal injuries and cause additional pain and damage.

Monitor the victim's vital signs and provide reassurance and support during transport to the medical facility.

Understanding how to assess and manage musculoskeletal injuries is essential for providing effective first aid and preventing further complications. Proper splinting techniques help immobilize injured limbs and reduce pain and discomfort.

When transporting victims with musculoskeletal injuries, it's important to prioritize their safety and well-being to ensure they receive timely and appropriate medical care.

CHAPTER NINE

Medical Emergencies
Signs and Symptoms of Common Medical Emergencies:

Heart Attack: Symptoms include chest pain or discomfort, pain or discomfort in the arms, back, neck, jaw, or stomach, shortness of breath, nausea, lightheadedness, and cold sweats.

Stroke: Signs may include sudden weakness or numbness of the face, arm, or leg, especially on one side of the body, confusion, trouble speaking or understanding speech, vision problems, severe headache, and difficulty walking.

Diabetic Emergencies:

Hypoglycemia (low blood sugar): Symptoms include shakiness, dizziness, sweating, confusion, irritability, hunger, weakness, and rapid heartbeat.

Hyperglycemia (high blood sugar): Symptoms include increased thirst, frequent urination, fatigue, nausea, vomiting, abdominal pain, shortness of breath, and fruity-smelling breath.

Initial First Aid Interventions for Medical Emergencies:

- Heart Attack:

1. Have the person sit or lie down in a comfortable position.

2. Loosen tight clothing and reassure the person.

3. If the person is conscious and not allergic to aspirin, have them chew and swallow a regular aspirin (325 mg) to help prevent blood clotting.

4. Monitor the person's vital signs and be prepared to administer CPR if necessary.

- Stroke:

1. Assess the person's level of consciousness and ability to speak or move.

2. Keep the person in a comfortable and supported position and reassure them.

3. Call emergency services immediately and provide details of the person's symptoms and any relevant medical history.

4. Do not give the person anything to eat or drink, as they may have difficulty swallowing.

- Diabetic Emergencies:

- Hypoglycemia:

1. Give the person a fast-acting carbohydrate such as fruit juice, glucose gel, or candy.

2. If the person is conscious, wait for symptoms to improve and then provide a snack or meal containing protein and carbohydrates.

3. If the person loses consciousness, place them in the recovery position and call for emergency medical assistance.

- Hyperglycemia:

1. Encourage the person to drink water to help flush excess glucose from their system.

2. Monitor the person's blood sugar levels if possible and seek medical advice if necessary.

Calling Emergency Medical Services (EMS) and Providing Essential Information

Dial the emergency number (e.g., 911) immediately to request assistance.

Provide the dispatcher with essential information, including the nature of the medical emergency, the location of the victim, any known medical conditions or allergies, and the current condition of the victim.

Stay on the line with the dispatcher and follow any instructions provided until help arrives.

If possible, designate someone to meet emergency responders and guide them to the location of the victim.

Getting the understanding of the signs and symptoms of common medical emergencies and knowing how to administer initial first aid interventions can help stabilize the victim and improve their chances of recovery. Promptly calling emergency services and providing essential information ensures that the victim receives timely and appropriate medical care.

CHAPTER TEN

Environmental Emergencies Recognition and Treatment of Heat-Related Illnesses (Heat Exhaustion, Heatstroke):

- Heat Exhaustion:

- Symptoms include heavy sweating, weakness, dizziness, nausea, headache, muscle cramps, and fainting.

- Move the person to a cooler environment, encourage them to rest, and offer cool fluids to drink.

- Loosen or remove tight clothing and apply cool, wet cloths to the skin to help lower body temperature.

- Monitor the person's condition and seek medical attention if symptoms worsen or persist.

- Heatstroke:

- Symptoms include high body temperature (above 103°F or 40°C), hot and dry skin, rapid pulse, throbbing headache, confusion, nausea, and unconsciousness.

- Call emergency services immediately and move the person to a cooler area.

- Remove excess clothing and use cool water or ice packs to lower body temperature.

- Continuously monitor the person's vital signs and provide supportive care until medical help arrives.

Hypothermia and Frostbite
Prevention and First Aid Measures:

- Hypothermia:

- Hypothermia occurs when the body loses heat faster than it can produce it, causing dangerously low body temperatures.

- Symptoms include shivering, confusion, slurred speech, shallow breathing, weak pulse, and loss of coordination.

- Move the person to a warm environment, remove wet clothing, and wrap them in blankets or warm clothing.

- Provide warm, non-alcoholic beverages and monitor the person's vital signs until medical help arrives.

- Frostbite:

- Frostbite occurs when skin and underlying tissues freeze due to exposure to cold temperatures.

- Symptoms include numbness, tingling, pain, pale or white skin, and stiff or waxy texture of the affected area.

- Immediately move the person to a warmer environment and remove wet clothing.

- Thaw the affected area gradually using warm (not hot) water or body heat.

- Do not rub the affected area or use direct heat sources, as this can cause further damage.

- Seek medical attention for severe frostbite or if symptoms do not improve.

Dealing with Altitude Sickness and Allergic Reactions

- Altitude Sickness:

- Altitude sickness can occur when ascending to high altitudes too quickly, leading to symptoms such as headache, nausea, dizziness, fatigue, and shortness of breath.

 - Descend to a lower altitude if symptoms are severe or persist.

- Rest, hydrate, and avoid alcohol and strenuous activity until symptoms improve.

- Consider using supplemental oxygen or medication to alleviate symptoms as needed.

- Allergic Reactions:

 - Allergic reactions can range from mild itching and hives to severe anaphylaxis, which can be life-threatening.

- Administer epinephrine (if available) immediately for severe allergic reactions.

- Call emergency services and seek medical attention promptly.

- Monitor the person's airway, breathing, and circulation and be prepared to perform CPR if necessary.

Understanding the recognition and treatment of environmental emergencies is crucial for ensuring the safety and well-being of individuals exposed to extreme environmental conditions.

Prompt intervention and appropriate first aid measures can help mitigate the effects of heat-related illnesses, hypothermia, frostbite, altitude sickness, and allergic reactions, improving outcomes and reducing the risk of complications.

CHAPTER ELEVEN

Child and Infant First Aid

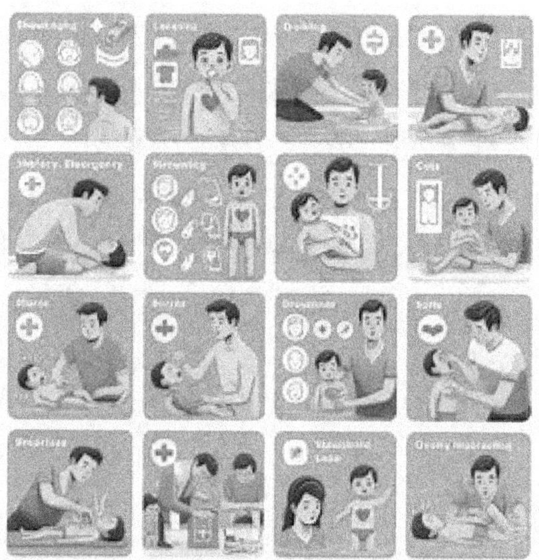

Special Considerations for Pediatric Emergencies:

Children and infants have unique anatomical and physiological differences compared to adults, requiring special considerations in first aid.

Children have proportionally larger heads, smaller airways, and higher metabolic rates than adults, which can affect their response to injuries and illnesses.

Recognizing and responding to pediatric emergencies requires knowledge of age-appropriate vital signs, normal developmental milestones, and common childhood illnesses and injuries.

CPR and Choking Relief Techniques for Infants and Children

CPR for Infants:

Place the infant on a firm surface and begin CPR by giving 30 chest compressions, using two fingers in the center of the chest just below the nipple line.

After 30 compressions, give two gentle breaths into the infant's mouth and nose, making sure to watch for chest rise.

Continue cycles of 30 compressions and two breaths at a rate of about 100-120 compressions per minute until help arrives or the infant begins to breathe spontaneously.

CPR for Children:

For children older than 1 year, use the heel of one hand to give chest compressions at a depth of about one-third the depth of the chest.

Give 30 chest compressions followed by two breaths into the child's mouth.

Continue CPR cycles until help arrives or the child begins to breathe on their own.

Choking Relief Techniques:

For infants younger than 1 year, administer back blows and chest thrusts to dislodge the obstruction.

For children older than 1 year, use abdominal thrusts (Heimlich maneuver) to clear the airway obstruction.

Perform these maneuvers until the object is expelled or the child becomes unconscious.

Common Childhood Emergencies and Their Management:

Febrile Seizures: Keep the child safe by laying them on their side and removing any nearby objects. Monitor their breathing and protect them from injury until the seizure stops.

Allergic Reactions: Administer epinephrine if the child has a known severe allergy. Call emergency services and seek medical attention immediately.

Burns: Cool the burned area with cool (not cold) water for at least 10 minutes. Cover the burn with a clean, dry cloth and seek medical attention if the burn is severe.

Poisoning: Call poison control immediately for guidance. Do not induce vomiting unless instructed by a healthcare professional. Keep any suspected poisons and containers for identification.

Understanding and being prepared to respond to pediatric emergencies is essential for caregivers and anyone who interacts with children regularly.

By knowing how to administer CPR and choking relief techniques specific to infants and children, as well as being familiar with common childhood emergencies and their management, individuals can help ensure the safety and well-being of young ones in emergency situations.

Regular training and practice in pediatric first aid techniques are recommended to maintain proficiency and confidence in responding to pediatric emergencies.

CHAPTER TWELVE

Psychological First Aid
Recognizing Signs of Emotional Distress and Trauma

Emotional distress and trauma can manifest in various ways, including;

- Intense fear, sadness, or anxiety

- Disorientation or confusion

- Withdrawal from social interactions

- Changes in behavior or mood

- Difficulty concentrating or making decisions

- Flashbacks or intrusive memories of traumatic events

- It's important to recognize that everyone responds differently to stress and trauma, and signs of distress may vary among individuals.

Providing Support and Reassurance to Victims

- Create a safe and supportive environment where the individual feels comfortable expressing their emotions and experiences.

- Listen actively and empathetically without judgment. Allow the individual to share their feelings and experiences at their own pace.

- Offer validation and reassurance by acknowledging their emotions and experiences as valid and understandable reactions to the situation.

- Use calming and supportive language to convey empathy and understanding. Avoid minimizing or dismissing the individual's feelings or experiences.

- Encourage self-care activities such as deep breathing, mindfulness, and engaging in activities that bring comfort and relaxation.

Referral and Follow-up Resources for Mental Health Support

- Provide information about local mental health resources, including crisis hotlines, counseling services, support groups, and community organizations that offer mental health support.

- Offer to assist the individual in connecting with mental health professionals or support services if needed.

- Encourage the individual to prioritize self-care and seek professional help if they continue to experience significant distress or impairment in functioning.

- Follow up with the individual periodically to check on their well-being and offer ongoing support and encouragement.

- Remind the individual that seeking help for mental health concerns is a sign of strength and resilience, and that they are not alone in their struggles.

Steps for Administering Psychological First Aid

Assessment: Observe the individual's behavior, emotions, and verbal cues to assess their level of distress and identify signs of trauma or emotional struggle.

Establish Rapport: Build rapport and trust by expressing empathy, actively listening, and validating the individual's experiences and feelings.

Provide Emotional Support: Offer emotional support and reassurance by acknowledging the individual's emotions and providing validation and empathy.

Offer Practical Assistance: Offer practical assistance or resources to help meet the individual's immediate needs and address any concerns or challenges they may be facing.

Encourage Self-care: Encourage the individual to engage in self-care activities and coping strategies to manage stress and promote emotional well-being.

Provide Information: Provide information about available mental health resources and support services, and assist the individual in accessing appropriate resources if needed.

Follow Up: Follow up with the individual to check on their well-being, offer ongoing support, and ensure they are connected with the necessary resources for continued support and care.

Recognizing signs of emotional distress and trauma, providing compassionate support and reassurance, and connecting individuals with appropriate mental health resources, psychological first aid can help promote resilience and recovery in the aftermath of stressful or traumatic events.

9 798884 615434